EPI Diet Food List

A Guide to Balanced Eating for Improved
Digestive Function

McDonnell B. Young

Table of Contents

Introduction   5

    Overview of Exocrine Pancreatic Insufficiency   8

    Importance of Diet in Managing EPI   11

    How to Use This Book   14

Chapter 1: Understanding EPI   17

    What is Exocrine Pancreatic Insufficiency?   17

    Symptoms and Diagnosis   20

    Treatment Options and Lifestyle Adjustments   23

Chapter 2: Nutritional Fundamentals for EPI   26

    Macronutrients: Balancing Fats, Proteins, and Carbohydrates   26

    Micronutrients: Vitamins and Minerals   29

    Importance of Hydration   32

Chapter 3: Foods to Eat   35

    Lean Proteins   35

    LowFat Dairy Alternatives   40

    Whole Grains   44

    Fruits and Vegetables   51

    Pancreatic EnzymeFriendly Snacks   57

Chapter 4: Foods to Avoid   61

    HighFat Foods   61

    DifficulttoDigest Grains   65

    Raw Fruits and Vegetables   71

    Sugary Foods and Drinks   76

    Alcoholic Beverages   81

Chapter 5: Meal Planning and Recipes   87

Breakfast Ideas ... 87

Lunch Ideas ... 91

Dinner Ideas ... 97

Snacks and Desserts ... 100

Conclusion ... **107**

Introduction

In the charming but bustling town of Maple Grove, there lived a kindly baker named Sarah who was famous for her wholesome breads and delectable pastries. Her little bakery, "Sarah's Sweets," was a hub of warmth and delicious aromas, drawing locals and tourists alike. However, beneath her cheerful demeanor, Sarah battled a challenging condition—Exocrine Pancreatic Insufficiency (EPI).

Sarah's journey with EPI began with confusion and discomfort. She faced numerous symptoms that made day-to-day life difficult: digestive upset, nutrient malabsorption, and a constant fatigue that seemed to overshadow her passion for baking. Each meal became a game of guessing and checking, which foods her body could handle and which would leave her feeling unwell.

Her turning point came when she discovered the "EPI Diet Food List Guide." Initially skeptical, Sarah decided to give it a chance, hoping to find a solution to manage her symptoms better. The guide was more than a mere list of foods; it was a comprehensive resource that explained the intricacies of EPI, the importance of diet management, and detailed lists of what to eat and what to avoid.

With the guide in hand, Sarah learned how to choose lean proteins that were easier on her pancreas, incorporate low-fat dairy alternatives that didn't cause distress, and select whole grains that provided her with energy without the discomfort. She discovered new ways to prepare her meals that maintained nutritional content without compromising taste.

Inspired by her newfound knowledge, Sarah began experimenting in her bakery. She replaced traditional ingredients with EPI-friendly alternatives, creating breads that were just as fluffy and pastries just as sweet, but much kinder to her system. Her bakery evolved to include a special section labeled "EPI-friendly," featuring all the new recipes she had perfected.

Word spread quickly through Maple Grove. Soon, Sarah's Sweets became a sanctuary not just for food lovers but also for those with EPI and other digestive disorders. Sarah shared her story with every curious customer, explaining how the "EPI Diet Food List Guide" had transformed her life and bakery.

One afternoon, a young woman named Elise walked into Sarah's Sweets. She looked around timidly, her expression one of someone long used to dietary restrictions. Sarah approached her with a comforting smile and they started talking. Elise shared her own struggles with EPI, her voice tinged with the frustration of countless disappointing meals and ongoing health issues.

With a gentle enthusiasm, Sarah recommended the "EPI Diet Food List Guide." She told Elise how it not only educated her about safe and harmful foods but also empowered her to make informed dietary choices that significantly alleviated her symptoms. "This isn't just a book," Sarah explained, "it's a gateway to a better, healthier life, even with EPI."

Elise, moved by Sarah's story and the delicious samples from the EPI-friendly section, decided to purchase the guide. As she left the bakery, guide tucked under her arm, there was a hopeful spring in her step—a feeling that, perhaps, this was the beginning of a better phase in her life.

Sarah watched Elise walk away, feeling a profound sense of fulfillment. The "EPI Diet Food List Guide" had not only changed her life; it was now set to change the lives of many others. In her heart, Sarah knew that every person struggling with EPI deserved to experience this transformation, to enjoy food without fear or pain, just as she had.

Through her bakery and her story, Sarah continued to advocate for the guide, a beacon of hope in the quaint town of Maple Grove, reminding everyone why they should consider this life-altering resource.

Overview of Exocrine Pancreatic Insufficiency

Exocrine Pancreatic Insufficiency (EPI) is a condition that occurs when the pancreas fails to produce enough of the enzymes necessary for proper digestion of foods. This deficiency can lead to malabsorption of nutrients, as the enzymes typically break down fats, proteins, and carbohydrates. People with EPI often experience symptoms such as weight loss, diarrhea, and steatorrhea, which is the presence of excess fat in the stools. This can result in nutritional deficiencies and a host of related health issues if not managed effectively.

The management of EPI typically involves a combination of enzyme replacement therapy and dietary adjustments to reduce symptoms and improve nutrient absorption. Enzyme supplements are usually taken with meals to help mimic the natural process of digestion. However, the dietary component is equally crucial as it directly influences the effectiveness of enzyme supplementation and overall digestive comfort.

In terms of dietary adjustments, individuals with EPI are advised to modify their intake of fats, as the pancreas plays a crucial role in fat digestion. High-fat foods can exacerbate symptoms and lead to discomfort. Instead, a diet low in fat and rich in easily digestible foods is recommended. This includes lean proteins, such as chicken and turkey, which provide necessary nutrients without overwhelming the digestive system.

Carbohydrates also need careful management, though they are generally easier to digest. Whole grains like oats and brown rice are beneficial as they provide energy and are less likely to cause digestive issues. However, fibrous foods can sometimes trigger symptoms, so the fiber intake must be tailored according to individual tolerance levels.

Fruits and vegetables are essential for their vitamins and minerals but should be consumed cooked rather than raw to ease digestion. Cooking helps break down some of the fibers and complex sugars in these foods, making them more digestible. Individuals should focus on low-fiber options to prevent aggravating EPI symptoms.

Aside from macronutrients, attention should also be given to the overall preparation and frequency of meals. Small, frequent meals can help manage the workload of the compromised pancreas more effectively than larger, more sporadic eating sessions. This approach not only aids in digestion but also helps maintain steady energy levels throughout the day.

Lastly, the relationship between diet and EPI is dynamic and individualized. What works for one person may not work for another, hence the importance of close monitoring and adjustments based on personal experiences and symptoms.

Consulting with a healthcare provider or a dietitian who specializes in EPI can provide guidance tailored to individual needs and help manage the condition more effectively through diet and lifestyle changes. This careful management can significantly improve quality of life for those affected by EPI.

Importance of Diet in Managing EPI

Diet plays a crucial role in managing Exocrine Pancreatic Insufficiency (EPI), a condition where the pancreas fails to produce sufficient digestive enzymes. This deficiency hampers the body's ability to break down foods, especially fats, which can lead to nutrient malabsorption and a host of digestive symptoms. Proper dietary management can significantly alleviate these symptoms by aiding the digestive process and ensuring that nutrients are more effectively absorbed.

For individuals with EPI, consuming easily digestible foods that are low in fat is essential. The pancreas of an EPI patient struggles with the digestion of fats, which can lead to unpleasant symptoms like steatorrhea, where fats are poorly absorbed and lead to fatty, oily stools. Adapting a diet that focuses on lean proteins, low-fat dairy alternatives, and cooked vegetables can help minimize these symptoms. Foods like grilled chicken, low-fat yogurts, and steamed vegetables become staples in their meals, providing necessary nutrients without overburdening the pancreas.

Carbohydrates also need careful management, though they are generally easier to digest. Opting for whole grains like oats and brown rice provides the energy EPI patients need without the risk of aggravating symptoms. These choices are crucial as they ensure a steady supply of energy throughout the day, which is essential because malabsorption can often lead to fatigue and weight loss.

However, it is important to avoid high-fiber options as they can be difficult to digest and may exacerbate symptoms.

Fruits and vegetables are also integral to the EPI diet but should be consumed with care. Raw fruits and vegetables can be challenging to digest; therefore, cooking or steaming them can make it easier for the gut to process. Low-fiber fruits like bananas and melons are recommended as they are gentler on the digestive system. These provide vital vitamins and antioxidants which are crucial for overall health, particularly for individuals battling chronic conditions like EPI.

In addition to what foods to eat, understanding which foods to avoid is equally important. Foods high in fat, such as fried foods and full-fat dairy products, should be strictly limited as they can significantly increase gastrointestinal distress. Similarly, alcoholic beverages and caffeinated drinks should be avoided as they can stimulate the digestive tract in ways that exacerbate symptoms, making management of EPI more challenging.

Supplemental enzymes are often a necessary part of managing EPI, as they help break down fats, proteins, and carbohydrates, facilitating better absorption. These supplements are typically taken with meals and snacks based on the amount of macronutrients consumed. This therapeutic approach is tailored to individual needs and can vary significantly from one person to another depending on the severity of their enzyme deficiency.

Maintaining a balanced diet while managing EPI is not just about symptom control; it's about enhancing the quality of life. Eating the right foods can help individuals feel more energetic and less burdened by their condition. The EPI diet food list serves as a comprehensive guide to making informed food choices that support digestive health and overall wellbeing. With careful planning and adjustments, those with EPI can lead a healthy and active life, minimizing the impact of their condition on their daily activities.

How to Use This Book

Navigating through the complexities of Exocrine Pancreatic Insufficiency (EPI) can be daunting, especially when it comes to dietary management. This book is designed to serve as a reliable companion in your journey to understanding and adapting to an EPI-friendly diet. It offers a structured approach, beginning with detailed explanations of EPI and its effects on digestion and nutrient absorption. By thoroughly understanding your condition, you can make more informed decisions about the foods you eat, which is crucial in managing symptoms and maintaining overall health.

The main section of the book contains comprehensive lists of foods that are recommended for individuals with EPI, as well as those that should be avoided. These lists are not merely enumerations but are accompanied by explanations on why certain foods might aggravate symptoms or how others can be beneficial. This detailed guidance is aimed at helping you make choices that can prevent discomfort and improve your digestive health. The book stresses the importance of lean proteins, low-fat cooking methods, and how to incorporate necessary vitamins and minerals through both food and supplements.

To make dietary management more practical, the book includes tips on how to read food labels, which is an essential skill for avoiding hidden sources of fats and sugars that can exacerbate

EPI. It also provides advice on meal planning and preparation, which can help you maintain a balanced diet without feeling overwhelmed. Techniques for cooking and food preparation are discussed to ensure that meals are not only safe but also appealing and flavorful.

Adopting any new diet is challenging, and the transition to an EPI-friendly diet is no exception. The book offers strategies for gradual dietary changes, allowing your body to adjust without causing undue stress. It encourages starting with small, manageable adjustments and gradually incorporating more changes as you become more comfortable with your new diet. This gradual approach helps mitigate the risk of digestive distress and makes the transition smoother and more sustainable.

Social eating and dining out can be particularly challenging for those managing EPI. The guide provides practical advice on how to navigate restaurants and social gatherings, including what questions to ask and how to make safe choices while dining out. This information is crucial for maintaining a social life and enjoying meals out without fear of triggering symptoms.

For ongoing support and adaptation, the book suggests keeping a food diary to track what you eat and how it affects your symptoms. This can be a powerful tool for identifying triggers and fine-tuning your diet. Over time, this tracking can help you recognize patterns and make necessary adjustments to your eating habits.

Finally, the book emphasizes the importance of regular consultations with healthcare professionals who can provide support and guidance tailored to your specific needs. Dietitians, nutritionists, and your medical team can offer insights and adjustments to ensure that your diet continues to support your health without compromising your quality of life. By using this book as a guide and collaborating with healthcare providers, you can effectively manage your EPI and lead a healthier, more comfortable life.

Chapter 1: Understanding EPI

What is Exocrine Pancreatic Insufficiency?

Exocrine Pancreatic Insufficiency (EPI) is a condition characterized by the inadequate production and secretion of pancreatic enzymes, which are crucial for the digestion of nutrients in the small intestine. The pancreas, a vital organ located behind the stomach, plays a significant role in digestion by producing enzymes that break down fats, proteins, and carbohydrates. In individuals with EPI, the pancreas fails to produce enough of these enzymes, leading to difficulties in digesting food and absorbing essential nutrients.

The deficiency in pancreatic enzymes results in several gastrointestinal symptoms, which include steatorrhea (fatty stools), weight loss, bloating, and abdominal pain. These symptoms arise because undigested food, especially fats, remains in the intestines, causing discomfort and nutritional deficiencies. The severity of symptoms can vary depending on how much enzyme production is compromised and can fluctuate over time with changes in diet and health status.

EPI can occur as a result of various underlying conditions that affect the pancreas. Chronic pancreatitis, cystic fibrosis, pancreatic cancer, and surgeries involving the pancreas are common causes. Each of these conditions can lead to the destruction or blocking of pancreatic tissue, thereby reducing enzyme output. It is also possible for EPI to develop without a clear underlying pancreatic disease, though this is less common.

The management of EPI primarily involves the replacement of pancreatic enzymes using supplemental enzymes, which are taken with meals to aid in the digestion of food. This treatment helps to reduce gastrointestinal symptoms and improve nutrient absorption. However, managing EPI goes beyond just enzyme replacement; dietary adjustments play a crucial role in alleviating symptoms and ensuring adequate nutrition.

An EPI-specific diet typically focuses on reducing fat intake to lower the digestive burden on the pancreas while ensuring a balanced intake of proteins and carbohydrates. It also emphasizes the importance of eating smaller, more frequent meals to facilitate easier digestion and absorption of nutrients. Foods that are easy to digest and less likely to cause irritation or discomfort are prioritized.

In addition to dietary management, individuals with EPI need to monitor their intake of fat-soluble vitamins (A, D, E, and K), as their absorption can be particularly affected. Supplements might be necessary to correct these deficiencies. Maintaining a balanced diet rich in nutrients, while adhering to the guidelines for fat and fiber intake, helps prevent the common complications associated with malabsorption in EPI.

Understanding EPI and its dietary management is critical for anyone diagnosed with the condition. By adhering to a diet tailored for reduced pancreatic function and using enzyme supplements, individuals with EPI can lead healthier lives. Continuous consultation with healthcare professionals, including gastroenterologists and dietitians, is essential for effectively managing the condition and adapting to any changes in health status or dietary needs.

Symptoms and Diagnosis

Exocrine Pancreatic Insufficiency (EPI) is a condition where the pancreas does not produce enough of the enzymes necessary for digesting foods, particularly fats, proteins, and carbohydrates. This deficiency can lead to a variety of gastrointestinal symptoms that often prompt individuals to seek medical advice. The most common symptoms include steatorrhea, which is the presence of excess fat in the stool, making the stool oily, foul-smelling, and difficult to flush. Patients might also experience weight loss, not due to a lack of eating, but because their bodies cannot absorb the nutrients from the food they consume.

Other symptoms that are frequently reported include abdominal pain and cramping, which are typically more pronounced after eating as the undigested food passes through the digestive tract. Diarrhea and increased bowel movements are common due to the rapid transit of food through the intestines. These symptoms can lead to further complications such as vitamin and mineral deficiencies, particularly of the fat-soluble vitamins A, D, E, and K, which require adequate pancreatic enzymes for absorption.

Diagnosing EPI can be challenging because its symptoms often overlap with those of other gastrointestinal disorders such as irritable bowel syndrome, celiac disease, and Crohn's disease. Generally, the diagnosis begins with a detailed medical history and a physical examination. Doctors look for key signs like unexplained weight loss and chronic diarrhea in combination with the medical history that suggests malabsorption or digestive problems.

To confirm a diagnosis of EPI, several tests may be used. The most direct test is the measurement of the elastase enzyme in a stool sample. Pancreatic elastase is an enzyme produced only by the pancreas, and its concentration in stool reflects pancreatic function. Low levels of fecal elastase suggest EPI. This test is particularly advantageous because it is non-invasive and highly specific, although it does not measure all aspects of pancreatic function.

Other tests might include blood tests to check for nutrient deficiencies that are common in EPI, such as fat-soluble vitamins and essential fatty acids. Imaging tests like a computed tomography (CT) scan or magnetic resonance imaging (MRI) of the abdomen might be conducted to check for structural problems in the pancreas and surrounding tissues. These tests help rule out other conditions that might mimic EPI, such as pancreatic tumors or cysts.

In some cases, more specialized tests, such as the secretin stimulation test, are conducted. This test involves administering a hormone that stimulates the pancreas to secrete its digestive enzymes and then measuring the output of pancreatic juice. It's more invasive and generally used if the diagnosis remains uncertain or if further detail on pancreatic function is necessary.

Management of EPI typically involves dietary adjustments and enzyme replacement therapy, which is crucial to improving quality of life. Patients are advised to follow a diet low in fats and fibrous materials and may be prescribed pancreatic enzyme replacement therapy to aid digestion. Regular follow-up with healthcare providers ensures that enzyme dosage and diet can be adjusted based on symptoms, promoting optimal digestion and nutrient absorption. Thus, understanding the symptoms and getting an accurate diagnosis are essential first steps in managing and living with EPI effectively.

Treatment Options and Lifestyle Adjustments

Treating Exocrine Pancreatic Insufficiency (EPI) requires a multifaceted approach, combining medical interventions with lifestyle and dietary adjustments. One of the cornerstone treatments for EPI involves the use of pancreatic enzyme replacement therapy (PERT). These enzymes are crucial for the digestion and absorption of nutrients, particularly fats, proteins, and carbohydrates. Patients typically take these enzyme supplements with every meal and snack to aid in digestion and reduce symptoms such as steatorrhea, which is the excretion of abnormal quantities of fat with the feces owing to reduced absorption of fat by the intestine.

In addition to enzyme replacement, individuals with EPI often require fat-soluble vitamin supplements. Vitamins A, D, E, and K absorption can be particularly problematic due to the impaired digestion of fat. Supplementing these vitamins under the guidance of a healthcare provider is essential to prevent deficiencies and maintain overall health. Regular monitoring of vitamin levels through blood tests can help ensure that the supplementation is effective and adjusted as needed.

Dietary management is equally critical in treating EPI. A diet low in fats and rich in easily digestible foods can significantly alleviate symptoms and improve nutrient absorption. Patients are advised to consume small, frequent meals throughout the day instead of larger, heavier meals, which can overwhelm the digestive system. This method helps maximize nutrient absorption and minimize gastrointestinal discomfort.

Staying hydrated is important for overall digestive health, especially for those with EPI. Adequate fluid intake helps improve the digestion and movement of food through the intestines. It can also help manage or prevent some symptoms associated with EPI, such as constipation, which can exacerbate discomfort and impair nutrient absorption further.

Lifestyle adjustments play a supportive role in managing EPI effectively. Regular physical activity can stimulate digestion and help maintain a healthy weight, which is important as weight loss can be a concern for those with EPI due to malabsorption. Exercise doesn't need to be strenuous; even moderate activities like walking or swimming can be beneficial.

Avoiding alcohol and smoking is also advised for individuals with EPI. Both can exacerbate symptoms and further impair pancreatic function. Alcohol, in particular, can contribute to dehydration and nutrient depletion, while smoking has been linked to an increased risk of pancreatic diseases.

Finally, ongoing communication with healthcare providers is crucial for managing EPI. Regular check-ups allow for the monitoring of the condition and adjustments to treatment as necessary. As EPI can be a progressive condition, treatments and dietary needs may change over time, necessitating a flexible approach to management. Engaging with a dietitian who understands EPI can also provide invaluable support, offering tailored advice and helping individuals navigate the complexities of diet planning to improve quality of life.

Chapter 2: Nutritional Fundamentals for EPI

Macronutrients: Balancing Fats, Proteins, and Carbohydrates

For individuals with Exocrine Pancreatic Insufficiency (EPI), understanding and balancing macronutrients—fats, proteins, and carbohydrates—is crucial for effective dietary management. Since EPI affects the pancreas's ability to produce essential digestive enzymes, it is particularly important to adjust the intake of these macronutrients to minimize digestive distress and ensure adequate nutrient absorption.

Fats are often the most challenging macronutrient for individuals with EPI to digest due to insufficient pancreatic lipase, the enzyme necessary for breaking down fats. A high-fat meal can lead to uncomfortable symptoms such as bloating, gas, and diarrhea. Therefore, it is recommended to limit fat intake and opt for low-fat or fat-free options when possible. Including medium-chain triglycerides (MCTs) in the diet can be beneficial because they are more easily absorbed and do not require pancreatic enzymes for digestion.

Proteins are essential for tissue repair and immune function, making adequate protein intake critical for those with EPI. However, the ability to break down protein can be compromised in EPI, leading to malnutrition if not managed properly. Choosing lean sources of protein such as chicken, turkey, fish, and legumes can help, as they are generally easier to digest and less taxing on the pancreas. It is also important to prepare proteins in a way that makes them easier to digest, such as baking or poaching, rather than frying.

Carbohydrates should be approached with caution in an EPI diet. While they are a vital energy source, not all carbohydrates are created equal. Simple carbohydrates, such as those found in sugary foods and drinks, can cause a rapid increase in blood sugar levels, which is not ideal for overall health. Complex carbohydrates, found in foods like whole grains, vegetables, and fruits, are generally better as they provide fiber, which aids in digestion and helps maintain steady blood sugar levels.

Balancing these macronutrients involves not only choosing the right types of fats, proteins, and carbohydrates but also monitoring portion sizes and meal timing to optimize digestion and absorption. Eating smaller, more frequent meals can help manage the workload of the compromised pancreas, allowing it to handle the digestive process more efficiently and reduce symptoms.

Additionally, the use of pancreatic enzyme replacement therapy (PERT) can be crucial in helping to digest these macronutrients. Enzyme supplements should be taken with meals and snacks to aid in the breakdown of fats, proteins, and carbohydrates, thereby improving nutrient absorption and reducing gastrointestinal symptoms.

In conclusion, managing macronutrients is a delicate balance that requires careful planning and consideration for individuals with EPI. By understanding the roles and digestion processes of fats, proteins, and carbohydrates, and adapting their intake accordingly, those with EPI can significantly improve their nutritional status and quality of life. Regular consultations with healthcare professionals and dietitians who specialize in digestive disorders can provide further personalized guidance and adjustments to the diet.

Micronutrients: Vitamins and Minerals

In managing Exocrine Pancreatic Insufficiency (EPI), a clear understanding of the role of micronutrients is crucial. EPI often leads to malabsorption, which can cause deficiencies in essential vitamins and minerals. These micronutrients are vital for numerous bodily functions, including immune system support, bone health, and the regulation of enzymes and hormones. Individuals with EPI need to pay particular attention to their intake of fat-soluble vitamins—A, D, E, and K—as their absorption is particularly affected by pancreatic enzyme insufficiency.

Vitamin A is essential for maintaining healthy vision, skin, and immune functions. For those with EPI, the absorption of this vitamin can be compromised, leading to deficiencies. It is beneficial to consume vitamin A from sources that are easier to digest and absorb, such as fortified foods or supplements prescribed by a healthcare provider. Similarly, vitamin D, which is crucial for bone health and calcium absorption, may also be deficient in individuals with EPI. Supplements or increased exposure to sunlight can help improve vitamin D levels, though it is important to monitor blood levels regularly under medical advice.

Vitamin E is an antioxidant that helps protect cells from damage and is important for the health of the skin, eyes, and immune system. Due to EPI affecting the digestion and absorption of fats, the intake of vitamin E needs to be monitored to prevent its deficiency. Nuts, seeds, and green leafy vegetables are good sources of vitamin E that may be included in a diet tailored for EPI, considering individual tolerance to these foods. Vitamin K is vital for blood clotting and bone health. Since its absorption depends on fat digestion, individuals with EPI may need to use supplements or consume vitamin K from sources that are easier to digest.

Beyond the fat-soluble vitamins, it is also important to ensure adequate intake of water-soluble vitamins, such as those from the B complex and vitamin C. These are less likely to be affected by EPI but are essential for overall health. B vitamins are crucial for energy production and neurological functions, and vitamin C is important for iron absorption and the maintenance of healthy skin and connective tissue.

Minerals such as calcium, magnesium, and zinc should also be monitored closely. Calcium is crucial for bone health and needs to be paired with vitamin D for proper absorption. Magnesium supports muscle and nerve functions and helps regulate blood sugar levels, which can be particularly important for people with EPI, who may have fluctuating blood sugar levels. Zinc is crucial for immune function and the healing of tissues, but like other minerals, its absorption can be impaired in EPI.

To manage these potential deficiencies, individuals with EPI are often advised to work with a dietitian who can recommend appropriate supplements and dietary adjustments. This approach ensures that their nutritional needs are met without exacerbating symptoms of EPI. Regular monitoring through blood tests can help adjust dietary plans and supplement doses to maintain optimal health while managing EPI effectively.

Importance of Hydration

Hydration plays a crucial role in overall health, but it is especially vital for individuals dealing with Exocrine Pancreatic Insufficiency (EPI). The condition can significantly affect digestion and nutrient absorption, making effective hydration a key component of dietary management. Water helps in the transport of nutrients and enzymes, which are critical for those with EPI, as their bodies struggle to break down and absorb nutrients from food.

When the pancreas is not functioning properly, as is the case with EPI, digestive enzymes are not adequately produced or delivered to the gut. This can lead to dehydration if not carefully managed, because fluids are essential in facilitating the digestive process and ensuring the smooth passage of food through the intestines. Proper hydration helps maintain the flow of pancreatic enzymes into the small intestine, enhancing digestion and the absorption of fats, proteins, and carbohydrates.

For those with EPI, dehydration can exacerbate digestive problems such as constipation and abdominal discomfort. Maintaining a consistent intake of fluids can prevent these issues by keeping the intestinal contents moving. This is particularly important since many EPI patients need to modify their dietary fiber intake to manage their symptoms, which can impact bowel regularity.

Water is not the only way to maintain hydration; other fluids like herbal teas and clear broths can also contribute effectively. However, individuals with EPI need to be cautious about the types of beverages they consume. Sugary drinks and alcoholic beverages can interfere with digestion and should be consumed minimally or avoided. Instead, opting for non-caffeinated, non-alcoholic, and low-sugar drinks can help maintain hydration without additional digestive stress.

Hydration also plays a role in the efficacy of pancreatic enzyme replacement therapy (PERT), commonly prescribed to manage EPI. These enzymes need a sufficiently hydrated environment to function optimally. Without enough fluids, the enzymes might not work as effectively, leading to malabsorption and malnutrition, despite proper medication adherence.

Moreover, hydration status can influence energy levels and cognitive function. For someone with EPI, whose nutrient absorption capabilities are compromised, staying well-hydrated is essential for maintaining energy throughout the day and supporting overall cognitive health. Chronic dehydration can lead to fatigue, which is already a common symptom in individuals with EPI due to malabsorption of essential nutrients.

In conclusion, maintaining adequate hydration is a foundational aspect of managing Exocrine Pancreatic Insufficiency. It supports digestive health, enhances the effectiveness of medications, and contributes to overall well-being. Those with EPI should aim to consume sufficient fluids throughout the day, heed the types of beverages they are ingesting, and consult with healthcare providers to tailor their hydration needs to their specific health circumstances.

Chapter 3: Foods to Eat

Lean Proteins

For individuals with Exocrine Pancreatic Insufficiency (EPI), incorporating lean proteins into their diet is crucial. Lean proteins are easier to digest and can be less taxing on the pancreas, which is important for those whose enzyme production is compromised. Below is a detailed table featuring a variety of lean protein dishes, each incorporating 15 different vegetables. The table provides ingredients, cooking instructions, nutritional information, serving sizes, and cooking times.

Dish Name	Ingredients	Instructions	Nutritional Information Per Serving	Serving Size	Cooking Time
Chicken Vegetable Stir-Fry	Chicken breast, broccoli,	1. Slice chicken and vegetables.	Calories: 350 Protein:	1 bowl	20 mins

	carrots, bell peppers (red, yellow), snow peas, spinach, zucchini, garlic, onion, asparagus, mushrooms, cabbage, celery, bamboo shoots, low-sodium soy sauce, olive oil	 2. Heat oil in a large pan. 3. Sauté garlic and onion until translucent. 4. Add chicken and vegetables; stir-fry until cooked.	27g Fat: 9g Carbs: 35g		

Turkey and Veggie Soup	Ground turkey, tomatoes, kale, spinach, carrots, onions, celery, garlic, green beans, peas, bell peppers, zucchini, yellow squash, parsley, chicken broth, black pepper	1. Brown turkey in a pot. 2. Add garlic, onions, and celery; cook until soft. 3. Add remaining ingredients and simmer until vegetables are tender.	Calories: 210 Protein: 18g Fat: 6g Carbs: 22g	1 bowl	30 mins

Grilled Fish with Salad	White fish (e.g., cod), lettuce, arugula, cherry tomatoes, cucumbers, radishes, carrots, bell peppers, red onions, avocado, lemon juice, olive oil, black pepper, dill	1. Season fish with lemon, dill, and pepper. 2. Grill until cooked through. 3. Toss all salad ingredients with olive oil and lemon juice.	Calories: 295 Protein: 25g Fat: 15g Carbs: 12g	1 serving	15 mins

These dishes are designed to be easy on the digestive system, providing ample nutrients without overloading the pancreas. The lean proteins offer substantial nourishment, while the variety of vegetables ensures a broad intake of vitamins and minerals essential for overall health. Each recipe is balanced to suit the dietary needs of those managing EPI, focusing on maximizing flavor without compromising nutritional value.

LowFat Dairy Alternatives

In managing Exocrine Pancreatic Insufficiency (EPI), selecting low-fat dairy alternatives is crucial due to the need to limit fat intake, which can exacerbate symptoms. Here is a comprehensive look at low-fat dairy alternatives, focusing on a detailed recipe that incorporates 15 different vegetables. This recipe is not only EPI-friendly but also nutritious and flavorful.

Recipe: Vegetable Medley with Coconut Yogurt Dressing

Ingredient	Quantity	Preparation
Carrots	2 medium	Peel and slice thinly
Zucchini	1 large	Dice
Yellow squash	1 large	Dice
Bell peppers (mixed colors)	3 (one of each color)	Seed and chop
Broccoli	1 head	Cut into florets
Cauliflower	1 head	Cut into florets
Spinach	2 cups	Fresh, washed

Kale	2 cups	Remove stems, chop
Peas	1 cup	Frozen, thawed
Green beans	1 cup	Trim and cut into one-inch pieces
Asparagus	1 bunch	Trim ends and cut into one-inch pieces
Mushrooms	1 cup	Sliced
Red onion	1 medium	Chop finely
Garlic	3 cloves	Minced
Cherry tomatoes	1 cup	Halve
Coconut yogurt	1 cup	Unsweetened
Lemon juice	2 tablespoons	Freshly squeezed
Dill	1 tablespoon	Fresh, chopped
Salt and pepper	To taste	—

Instructions:

1. Steam carrots, broccoli, cauliflower, green beans, and asparagus until tender-crisp, about 7-8 minutes.
2. In a large skillet, sauté red onion, garlic, bell peppers, zucchini, yellow squash, and mushrooms with a splash of water or vegetable broth for about 5 minutes, until softened.
3. Add steamed vegetables to the skillet and mix in peas, spinach, and kale. Cook until the greens are wilted, about 2 minutes.
4. Remove from heat and let cool slightly. Toss in cherry tomatoes.
5. In a separate bowl, mix coconut yogurt, lemon juice, dill, salt, and pepper to make the dressing.
6. Drizzle the dressing over the vegetable medley and toss to coat evenly.
7. Serve warm or at room temperature.

Nutritional Information:

- **Serving Size:** 1 cup
- **Calories:** 120
- **Total Fat:** 3g (Saturated Fat: 1g)
- **Cholesterol:** 0mg
- **Sodium:** 50mg
- **Total Carbohydrates:** 20g (Dietary Fiber: 6g, Sugars: 8g)
- **Protein:** 5g

Cooking Time: 20 minutes

This dish not only provides a wide array of nutrients from the variety of vegetables but also incorporates a dairy-free, low-fat alternative with the coconut yogurt dressing, making it ideal for those managing EPI and seeking to maintain a balanced, nutritious diet.

Whole Grains

When managing Exocrine Pancreatic Insufficiency (EPI), incorporating whole grains into the diet can be beneficial due to their nutrient density and fiber content, which help support digestive health. Here's a comprehensive guide to preparing a whole grain dish, specifically a hearty whole grain salad, featuring 15 different vegetables. This dish is designed to be nutritious, fiber-rich, and EPI-friendly, supporting digestion without overburdening the pancreas.

Ingredient	Quantity	Preparation	Nutritional Information per Serving	Serving Size	Cooking Time
Quinoa	1 cup	Rinse thoroughly	Calories: 222 Fiber: 5g Protein: 8g	1 cup	20 minutes

Chopped spinach	2 cups	Wash and chop	Calories: 14 Fiber: 1.6g Vitamin K: 483mcg	1/2 cup	-
Diced carrots	1 cup	Peel and dice	Calories: 52 Fiber: 3.6g Vitamin A: 21384 IU	1/4 cup	-
Sliced red bell peppers	1 cup	Core and slice	Calories: 19 Fiber: 1.5g Vitamin C: 95 mg	1/4 cup	-

Chopped broccoli	1 cup	Wash and chop into small florets	Calories: 31 Fiber: 2.4g Vitamin C: 81mg	1/4 cup	5 minutes
Diced cucumber	1 cup	Wash and dice without peeling	Calories: 16 Fiber: 0.5g	1/4 cup	-
Halved cherry tomatoes	1 cup	Wash and halve	Calories: 27 Fiber: 1.8g Vitamin C: 17mg	1/4 cup	-
Sliced zucchini	1 cup	Wash and slice	Calories: 19 	1/4 cup	-

			Fiber: 1.2g		
Shredded kale	1 cup	Wash and shred	Calories: 34 Fiber: 1.3g Vitamin C: 80.4 mg	1/4 cup	-
Corn kernels	1 cup	Boil if fresh, thaw if frozen	Calories: 125 Fiber: 3.6g Vitamin C: 6.2 mg	1/4 cup	5-7 minutes
Sliced mushrooms	1 cup	Wash and slice	Calories: 15 Fiber: 0.5g	1/4 cup	-

Chopped celery	1 cup	Wash and chop	Calories: 16 Fiber: 1.6g	1/4 cup	-
Peas	1 cup	Boil if fresh, thaw if frozen	Calories: 62 Fiber: 4g	1/4 cup	3 minutes
Chopped red onion	1/2 cup	Peel and chop finely	Calories: 32 Fiber: 0.7g	1/8 cup	-
Minced garlic	2 cloves	Peel and mince	Calories: 9 Fiber: 0.1g	1 clove	-
Olive oil	3 tablespoons	-	Calories: 119<br	1 tablespoon	-

			>Fat: 13.5g		
Lemon juice	2 tablespoons	Squeeze fresh lemons	Calories: 7 Vitamin C: 6.4mg	1 tablespoon	-
Salt and pepper	To taste	-	-	-	-

Instructions:

1. Start by cooking the quinoa according to package instructions; typically, this involves simmering in water for about 15-20 minutes until the grains become translucent and the spiral-like germ appears.
2. While the quinoa cooks, prepare the vegetables as described. For the broccoli and peas, briefly boil them to enhance their digestibility, which is particularly important for individuals with EPI.
3. In a large mixing bowl, combine the cooked quinoa and all the prepared vegetables. Drizzle with olive oil and lemon juice, then season with salt and pepper to taste.

Toss everything together to ensure the dressing and seasonings are evenly distributed.

4.   Allow the salad to sit for a few minutes before serving. This resting time lets the flavors meld together more harmoniously.

This whole grain salad offers a balanced meal with a variety of nutrients beneficial for managing EPI, including a good balance of fiber, vitamins, and a moderate amount of protein, all necessary for optimal digestive health.

Fruits and Vegetables

For individuals managing Exocrine Pancreatic Insufficiency (EPI), incorporating the right fruits and vegetables into their diet is crucial for ensuring they receive essential nutrients while avoiding digestive distress. Below is a detailed table featuring 15 vegetables that are beneficial for those with EPI. This table includes the vegetable name, instructions for preparation, nutritional information, recommended serving sizes, and approximate cooking times to optimize digestion and nutrient absorption.

Vegetable	Preparation Instructions	Nutritional Information (per 100g)	Serving Size	Cooking Time
Carrots	Peel and steam until tender. Can be mashed for easier digestion.	Calories: 41, Fiber: 2.8g, Vitamin A: 835µg	1/2 cup	10-15 min

Spinach	Steam lightly to retain nutrients but soften leaves. Serve warm.	Calories: 23, Fiber: 2.2g, Vitamin K: 483µg	1 cup	2-3 min
Pumpkin	Roast cubes with a touch of olive oil until soft.	Calories: 26, Fiber: 0.5g, Vitamin A: 8513 IU	1/2 cup	25-30 min
Zucchini	Slice and steam until tender. Can be pureed for soups.	Calories: 17, Fiber: 1g, Vitamin C: 17.9 mg	1/2 cup	5-7 min
Sweet potatoes	Bake or mash with a bit of	Calories: 86, Fiber: 3g,	1/2 cup	30-40 min

	cinnamon for flavor enhancem ent.	Vitamin A: 709 μg		
Beets	Boil or steam until tender. Peel and slice or puree.	Calories: 43, Fiber: 2.8g, Vitamin C: 4.9 mg	1/2 cup	30-40 min
Asparagus	Trim ends and steam lightly to maintain crispness and nutrients.	Calories: 20, Fiber: 2.1g, Vitamin K: 41.6μg	4-5 spears	4-5 min
Green beans	Steam or boil until they are tender. Serve	Calories: 31, Fiber: 2.7g, Vitamin C: 12.2 mg	1/2 cup	5-6 min

	whole or chopped.			
Broccoli	Steam until just tender to maximize nutrients and ease of digestion.	Calories: 34, Fiber: 2.6g, Vitamin C: 89.2 mg	1/2 cup	5-6 min
Butternut squash	Cube and roast or steam until soft. Can be pureed for soups or sauces.	Calories: 45, Fiber: 2g, Vitamin A: 532 μg	1/2 cup	25-30 min
Bell peppers	Steam or roast lightly to soften. Ideal for adding	Calories: 31, Fiber: 2.1g, Vitamin C: 127.7mg	1/2 cup	5-10 min

	flavor without fat.			
Cauliflower	Steam or roast until tender. Can be mashed or used in place of rice.	Calories: 25, Fiber: 2g, Vitamin C: 48.2 mg	1/2 cup	5-10 min
Peas	Steam lightly or boil to maintain sweetness and soft texture.	Calories: 81, Fiber: 5.1g, Vitamin C: 40 mg	1/2 cup	3-5 min
Brussels sprouts	Halve and steam or roast with minimal oil until tender.	Calories: 43, Fiber: 3.8g, Vitamin K: 177 µg	1/2 cup	6-8 min

Acorn squash	Halve and roast face down until flesh is tender. Can be scooped and served.	Calories: 40, Fiber: 1.5g, Vitamin A: 367 IU	1/2 cup	25-35 min

This table provides a useful guide for individuals with EPI to incorporate vegetables into their meals safely and deliciously, ensuring they receive the nutrients they need while managing their condition effectively.

Pancreatic EnzymeFriendly Snacks

Here is a detailed recipe for a 'Pancreatic Enzyme-Friendly Vegetable Quiche," which is suitable for individuals managing Exocrine Pancreatic Insufficiency (EPI). This recipe incorporates 15 different vegetables, providing a variety of nutrients while being gentle on the digestive system. The recipe also includes instructions, nutritional information, serving size, and cooking time in a comprehensive format.

Ingredient	Amount
Olive oil	1 tablespoon
Garlic, minced	2 cloves
Onion, chopped	1 medium
Red bell pepper, diced	1 medium
Green bell pepper, diced	1 medium
Zucchini, sliced	1 medium
Yellow squash, sliced	1 medium
Carrot, grated	1 large
Broccoli florets, chopped	1 cup

Cauliflower florets, chopped	1 cup
Spinach, chopped	1 cup
Mushrooms, sliced	1 cup
Cherry tomatoes, halved	1 cup
Asparagus, chopped	1 cup
Eggplant, diced	1 cup
Eggs	6 large
Low-fat milk	1 cup
Salt and pepper	To taste
Low-fat shredded cheese	1/2 cup

Instructions:

1. Preheat the oven to 375°F (190°C).
2. Heat olive oil in a large skillet over medium heat. Add garlic and onion, and sauté until translucent.

3. Add red and green bell peppers, zucchini, yellow squash, carrot, broccoli, cauliflower, and sauté for about 5 minutes until they are slightly soft.

4. Add spinach, mushrooms, cherry tomatoes, asparagus, and eggplant. Cook for another 5 minutes until all vegetables are tender.

5. In a large mixing bowl, whisk together eggs, low-fat milk, salt, and pepper.

6. Grease a pie dish or quiche pan. Spread the sautéed vegetables evenly across the bottom. Pour the egg mixture over the vegetables.

7. Sprinkle the top with low-fat shredded cheese.

8. Bake in the preheated oven for 35-40 minutes, or until the eggs are set and the top is golden brown.

Nutritional Information per serving:

- Calories: 150
- Protein: 9g
- Fat: 8g (2g saturated fat)
- Carbohydrates: 13g
- Fiber: 3g
- Sodium: 200mg

Serving Size: 1 slice (1/8 of quiche)

Cooking Time: 50 minutes (10 minutes prep time + 40 minutes cook time)

This quiche is rich in vegetables, providing a wide range of vitamins and minerals while being low in fat, which is crucial for those managing EPI. The protein from the eggs aids in sustaining energy levels and supporting tissue repair without putting excessive strain on the pancreas. This recipe is designed to be both nutritious and flavorful, making it a perfect snack or meal option for those on a pancreatic enzyme-friendly diet.

Chapter 4: Foods to Avoid

HighFat Foods

Creating a comprehensive guide on high-fat foods to avoid for those managing Exocrine Pancreatic Insufficiency (EPI) is crucial, as such foods can exacerbate symptoms and hinder effective digestion. Below is a detailed table that outlines specific high-fat vegetables, including their preparation methods, nutritional information, serving sizes, and cooking times. This information can help individuals with EPI make informed dietary choices to minimize discomfort and optimize health.

Vegetable	Preparation Method	Nutritional Information per Serving	Serving Size	Cooking Time
Avocado	Sliced raw	240 calories, 22g fat	1 medium	None
Olives (black)	Pitted and served whole	50 calories, 5g fat	10 olives	None

Coconut (shredded)	Used as topping	185 calories, 18g fat	2 tablespoons	None
Artichoke (hearts)	Marinated in oil	90 calories, 7g fat	3 pieces	None
Pumpkin seeds	Roasted with oil	71 calories, 6g fat	1 tablespoon	10 min
Sunflower seeds	Roasted	93 calories, 8g fat	1 tablespoon	10 min
Walnuts	Raw or toasted	185 calories, 18.5g fat	¼ cup	Optional
Cashews	Roasted with oil	165 calories, 13g fat	¼ cup	10-15 min
Almonds	Roasted	163 calories, 14g fat	¼ cup	10-15 min

Hazelnuts	Toasted	178 calories, 17g fat	¼ cup	10-15 min
Pine nuts	Toasted	191 calories, 19g fat	¼ cup	5-10 min
Pecans	Raw or toasted	196 calories, 20g fat	¼ cup	Optional
Brazil nuts	Raw or toasted	186 calories, 19g fat	¼ cup	Optional
Macadamia nuts	Raw or toasted	204 calories, 21.5g fat	¼ cup	Optional
Peanuts	Roasted with oil	166 calories, 14g fat	¼ cup	10-15 min

This table is designed to provide a clear overview of various high-fat vegetable sources that individuals with EPI should consider limiting or avoiding. By understanding the fat content and the ways these foods are typically prepared, those with EPI can better manage their symptoms and dietary intake. The cooking times are included to assist in preparation, though it's important to note that raw or minimal processing is often preferable to avoid adding extra fats through cooking methods such as roasting in oil.

DifficulttoDigest Grains

Creating a comprehensive guide about "Difficult-to-Digest Grains" in relation to an EPI diet requires understanding which grains may exacerbate symptoms for individuals with Exocrine Pancreatic Insufficiency. This guide will focus on common grains that are often harder to digest due to their high fiber content or complex structures, which can challenge an already compromised digestive system.

Here is a table detailing some typical grains to avoid, accompanied by a selection of 15 vegetables, providing ingredient details, instructions, nutritional information, serving size, and cooking time to facilitate an EPI-friendly diet:

Vegetable	Ingredients Needed	Cooking Instructions	Nutritional Information (per serving)	Serving Size	Cooking Time
Steamed Carrots	Carrots, water, salt	Peel carrots, slice, and	Calories: 55, Fat: 0.3g,	1 cup	10 mins

		steam until tender.	Fiber: 3.6g		
Mashed Potatoes	Potatoes, milk, butter	Boil peeled potatoes, mash with milk and butter.	Calories: 160, Fat: 6g, Fiber: 3g	1 cup	20 mins
Roasted Beets	Beets, olive oil, salt	Peel and slice beets, roast with olive oil until tender.	Calories: 75, Fat: 3.8g, Fiber: 3.4g	1 cup	45 mins
Boiled Spinach	Spinach, water, salt	Boil spinach leaves briefly	Calories: 7, Fat: 0.1g,	1 cup	5 mins

		until wilted.	Fiber: 0.7g		
Grilled Zucchini	Zucchini, olive oil, salt	Slice zucchini, grill with olive oil until tender.	Calories: 20, Fat: 1.7g, Fiber: 1g	1 cup	10 mins
Sautéed Kale	Kale, garlic, olive oil	Sauté kale and garlic in olive oil until tender.	Calories: 50, Fat: 2.9g, Fiber: 0.6g	1 cup	5 mins
Baked Squash	Squash, olive oil, salt	Slice squash, bake with olive oil until soft.	Calories: 76, Fat: 3.6g, Fiber: 5.7g	1 cup	35 mins

Steamed Broccoli	Broccoli, water, salt	Steam broccoli florets until tender.	Calories: 55, Fat: 0.6g, Fiber: 3.8g	1 cup	8 mins
Roasted Asparagus	Asparagus, olive oil, salt	Trim asparagus, roast with olive oil until crispy.	Calories: 20, Fat: 1.2g, Fiber: 2.1g	1 cup	15 mins
Baked Sweet Potatoes	Sweet potatoes, oil	Bake whole sweet potatoes until fork-tender.	Calories: 112, Fat: 0.1g, Fiber: 3.9g	1 medium	45 mins
Boiled Peas	Peas, water, salt	Boil peas until tender.	Calories: 62, Fat: 0.4g,	1 cup	8 mins

			Fiber: 4.8g		
Sautéed Mushrooms	Mushrooms, butter, garlic	Sauté sliced mushrooms and garlic in butter until browned.	Calories: 15, Fat: 0.2g, Fiber: 0.5g	1 cup	7 mins
Grilled Eggplant	Eggplant, olive oil, salt	Slice eggplant, grill with olive oil until tender.	Calories: 20, Fat: 0.1g, Fiber: 2.5g	1 cup	10 mins
Roasted Bell Peppers	Bell peppers, oil	Halve bell peppers, roast until	Calories: 51, Fat: 0.4g,	1 cup	25 mins

		skin blisters.	Fiber: 1.8g		
Steamed Cabbage	Cabbage, water, salt	Shred cabbage, steam until tender.	Calories: 17, Fat: 0.1g, Fiber: 2.2g	1 cup	12 mins

Each of these vegetables provides a healthy alternative to difficult-to-digest grains, offering essential nutrients while being easier on the digestive system for individuals managing EPI. This information is designed to help you incorporate a variety of vegetables into your diet safely and deliciously, contributing to overall digestive health and nutrient absorption.

Raw Fruits and Vegetables

For individuals managing Exocrine Pancreatic Insufficiency (EPI), consuming raw fruits and vegetables can pose a challenge. These foods often contain complex fibers that are difficult to digest for those with EPI, as their condition limits the production or activity of the digestive enzymes necessary to break down these fibers. This can lead to digestive distress, including bloating, gas, and abdominal pain. It's generally recommended to avoid or limit the consumption of raw produce and opt for cooked versions, which are easier to digest. Here's a comprehensive guide on how to prepare and serve 15 different vegetables in a way that's suitable for someone with EPI:

Vegetable	Preparation Instructions	Nutritional Information per Serving	Serving Size	Cooking Time
Carrots	Peel and steam until soft.	55 calories, 0.1g fat, 12.8g carbs	1 cup	10 mins

Spinach	Blanch to reduce oxalates and ease digestion.	7 calories, 0.1g fat, 1.1g carbs	1 cup	2 mins
Broccoli	Steam until tender to aid in easier digestion.	55 calories, 0.6g fat, 11g carbs	1 cup	5-7 mins
Zucchini	Steam or sauté until soft.	20 calories, 0.2g fat, 4.2g carbs	1 cup	5-7 mins
Pumpkin	Bake or steam until mushy.	30 calories, 0.1g fat, 8g carbs	1 cup	45 mins
Sweet potatoes	Boil or bake until soft.	112 calories, 0.1g fat, 26g carbs	1 cup	30 mins

Beets	Roast or boil until tender.	59 calories, 0.2g fat, 13g carbs	1 cup	45 mins
Cauliflower	Steam or bake until very soft.	25 calories, 0.1g fat, 5g carbs	1 cup	5-7 mins
Green beans	Steam or boil until soft.	44 calories, 0.1g fat, 10g carbs	1 cup	5 mins
Asparagus	Steam until soft and tender.	27 calories, 0.2g fat, 5.2g carbs	1 cup	4-5 mins
Brussels sprouts	Steam or roast until soft.	38 calories, 0.3g fat, 8g carbs	1 cup	6-8 mins
Butternut squash	Roast or steam	82 calories,	1 cup	45 mins

	until flesh is very soft and easily mashed.	0.2g fat, 21.5g carbs		
Peas	Boil or steam until very soft.	62 calories, 0.4g fat, 11g carbs	1 cup	5-7 mins
Tomatoes	Cook to reduce acidity and ease digestion.	32 calories, 0.2g fat, 7g carbs	1 cup	5 mins
Mushrooms	Cook thoroughly to break down tough cell walls.	15 calories, 0.2g fat, 2.3g carbs	1 cup	5-7 mins

These preparation methods help to soften the vegetables, making them more digestible and less likely to cause discomfort for individuals with EPI. By cooking these vegetables, you help in breaking down some of the fibers and complex carbohydrates, which can ease the digestive process in those lacking sufficient pancreatic enzymes.

Sugary Foods and Drinks

For individuals managing Exocrine Pancreatic Insufficiency (EPI), it's crucial to be mindful of the dietary choices, particularly avoiding sugary foods and drinks. These can exacerbate symptoms of EPI by stimulating the pancreas to release more digestive enzymes, which can be problematic when the pancreas is already compromised. Sugary items can also contribute to other health issues like blood sugar spikes, weight gain, and even diabetes, which can further complicate EPI management.

Here's a detailed table featuring a recipe that excludes sugary foods and drinks, focusing instead on a wholesome dish made from 15 different vegetables. This recipe provides a nutritious alternative that fits well within an EPI-friendly diet.

Ingredient	Amount	Preparation	Nutritional Information per Serving	Cooking Time
Zucchini	1 cup	Chopped	Calories: 20, Fat: 0.2g, Fiber: 1g	30 minutes

Carrots	1 cup	Diced	Calories: 41, Fat: 0.2g, Fiber: 2.8g	
Bell peppers (red and green)	1 cup	Sliced	Calories: 24, Fat: 0.2g, Fiber: 1.7g	
Eggplant	1 cup	Cubed	Calories: 20, Fat: 0.1g, Fiber: 2.5g	
Tomatoes	1 cup	Chopped	Calories: 32, Fat: 0.2g, Fiber: 2.2g	
Spinach	1 cup	Roughly chopped	Calories: 7, Fat: 0.1g,	

			Fiber: 0.7g	
Broccoli	1 cup	Florets	Calories: 31, Fat: 0.3g, Fiber: 2.4g	
Cauliflower	1 cup	Florets	Calories: 25, Fat: 0.1g, Fiber: 2g	
Asparagus	1 cup	Trimmed and cut into 1-inch pieces	Calories: 27, Fat: 0.2g, Fiber: 2.8g	
Sweet potatoes	1 cup	Peeled and diced	Calories: 114, Fat: 0.1g, Fiber: 3.3g	

Onions	1/2 cup	Finely chopped	Calories: 32, Fat: 0.1g, Fiber: 1.2g	
Garlic	2 cloves	Minced	Calories: 9, Fat: 0g, Fiber: 0.1g	
Mushrooms	1 cup	Sliced	Calories: 15, Fat: 0.2g, Fiber: 0.7g	
Green beans	1 cup	Trimmed	Calories: 31, Fat: 0.1g, Fiber: 2.7g	
Peas	1 cup	Shelled	Calories: 62, Fat: 0.4g,	

			Fiber: 4.4g	

Instructions:

1. Preheat your oven to 400°F (200°C).
2. Combine all the chopped and prepared vegetables in a large mixing bowl. Drizzle with olive oil and a pinch of salt, then toss to coat evenly.
3. Spread the vegetables on a baking sheet in a single layer.
4. Roast in the preheated oven for about 30 minutes, or until vegetables are tender and have caramelized edges, stirring halfway through.
5. Serve warm as a side dish or a main course for a fiber-rich, nutrient-packed meal.

Serving Size: This recipe yields approximately 4 servings, making it perfect for a family dinner.

This recipe avoids the use of any sugary components, focusing on the natural flavors and nutrients of the vegetables, making it ideal for those managing EPI. It provides a wholesome, satisfying meal that supports digestive health and overall wellness.

Alcoholic Beverages

For individuals managing Exocrine Pancreatic Insufficiency (EPI), careful dietary choices are crucial. One important recommendation is to avoid or significantly limit alcoholic beverages. Alcohol can exacerbate the symptoms of EPI by irritating the pancreas, increasing the demand for pancreatic enzymes, and potentially leading to further complications, including pancreatic flares. Here, instead of focusing on alcoholic beverages, we shift our attention to a healthier dietary choice, providing a detailed recipe for a nutrient-rich vegetable soup tailored for those with EPI. This soup avoids ingredients that could trigger symptoms and focuses on maximizing nutritional benefits.

EPI-Friendly Vegetable Soup Recipe

Ingredient	Quantity	Instruction	Nutritional Information per Serving	Serving Size	Cooking Time

Carrots	2 medium	Peel and chop finely	Rich in beta-carotene, fiber, vitamin K	1 cup	30 minutes
Celery	3 stalks	Chop finely	Low calories, provides fiber, vitamin C	1 cup	30 minutes
Broccoli	1 head	Chop into small florets	High in fiber, vitamin C and K, iron	1 cup	30 minutes
Spinach	2 cups	Rinse and chop	High in iron, magnesium, vitamins A, C, and E	1 cup	30 minutes

Zucchini	1 large	Dice	Low calorie, high in vitamin A, C, potassium	1 cup	30 minutes
Yellow squash	1 large	Dice	Contains magnesium, fiber, and folate	1 cup	30 minutes
Green beans	1 cup	Trim ends and chop	Good source of fiber, vitamins A, C, and K	1 cup	30 minutes
Bell peppers (red)	1 medium	Chop finely	High in antioxidants and	1 cup	30 minutes

			vitamins C, B6		
Sweet potatoes	1 medium	Peel and cube	Rich in fiber, vitamins A, C, and B6	1 cup	30 minutes
Tomatoes	2 large	Dice	Contains lycopene, vitamins C, potassium	1 cup	30 minutes
Garlic	3 cloves	Mince	Low calorie, boosts immunity	1 teaspoon	30 minutes
Onion	1 large	Chop finely	Provides fiber, vitamin	1 cup	30 minutes

			s C and B6		
Fresh ginger	2 inches	Peel and mince	Aids digestion, reduces nausea	1 tablespoon	30 minutes
Fresh turmeric	1 inch	Peel and mince	Anti-inflammatory, improves digestion	1 tablespoon	30 minutes
Cabbage	1/2 small head	Chop finely	High in vitamin C and K, improves digestion	1 cup	30 minutes

Instructions:

1. In a large pot, heat a tablespoon of olive oil over medium heat.
2. Add the garlic, onion, ginger, and turmeric. Sauté until the onions become translucent.
3. Add all the other vegetables to the pot, stirring to mix well.
4. Pour in enough water or a low-sodium vegetable broth to cover the vegetables.
5. Bring the soup to a boil, then reduce the heat and simmer for about 30 minutes until all vegetables are tender.
6. Season with a pinch of salt (optional) and pepper to taste.

Cooking Time: Total preparation and cooking time is approximately 40 minutes.

Serving Size: This recipe makes approximately 6 servings of 1 cup each.

Nutritional Information: Each serving provides a rich mix of vitamins, minerals, and fiber while being low in fat and calories, making it ideal for those managing EPI.

This soup serves as a comforting, nourishing meal that aligns with dietary recommendations for EPI, helping to avoid the triggers that alcoholic beverages may introduce.

Chapter 5: Meal Planning and Recipes

A. Oatmeal with Sliced Bananas and Almond Butter

Ingredients:
- Rolled oats: 1 cup
- Water or almond milk: 2 cups
- Banana: 1, sliced
- Almond butter: 1 tablespoon

Instructions:
1. Bring water or almond milk to a boil in a small pot.
2. Add rolled oats and reduce heat to a simmer, cooking for 10 minutes, stirring occasionally.
3. Once cooked, transfer to a bowl and top with sliced banana and a dollop of almond butter.

Nutritional Information:
- Calories: 380
- Protein: 10g

- Fat: 15g (low in saturated fat)
- Fiber: 6g

Serving Size:
- Makes 1 serving

Cooking Time:
- Total preparation and cooking time is approximately 15 minutes.

B. Scrambled Eggs with Spinach and Feta

Ingredients:
- Eggs: 2
- Fresh spinach: 1 cup, chopped
- Feta cheese: 1 ounce, crumbled
- Olive oil: 1 teaspoon

Instructions:
1. Heat olive oil in a non-stick skillet over medium heat.
2. Add fresh spinach and sauté until wilted, about 2 minutes.
3. Beat eggs in a bowl and pour over the spinach, stirring to combine.
4. Add crumbled feta and cook, stirring occasionally, until eggs are set, about 3-4 minutes.

Nutritional Information:
- Calories: 300
- Protein: 20g
- Fat: 22g (healthy fats from olive oil and feta)
- Fiber: 1g

Serving Size:
- Makes 1 serving

Cooking Time:
- Total preparation and cooking time is approximately 10 minutes.

C. Smoothie with Avocado, Blueberries, and Chia Seeds

Ingredients:
- Avocado: 1/2, peeled and pitted
- Blueberries: 1/2 cup, fresh or frozen
- Chia seeds: 1 tablespoon
- Almond milk or water: 1 cup

Instructions:
1. Combine all ingredients in a blender.
2. Blend on high until smooth.

Nutritional Information:

- Calories: 250
- Protein: 4g
- Fat: 18g (healthy fats from avocado and chia seeds)
- Fiber: 9g

Serving Size:

- Makes 1 serving

Cooking Time:

- Total preparation and blending time is approximately 5 minutes.

Lunch Ideas

Meal planning is an essential tool for managing Exocrine Pancreatic Insufficiency (EPI), ensuring that every meal not only tastes good but also aligns with dietary needs to avoid exacerbating symptoms. Here, we focus on lunch, often a challenging meal for those trying to balance work, life, and dietary restrictions. Below are two lunch ideas, including all necessary details like ingredients, instructions, nutritional information, serving sizes, and cooking times.

1. Grilled Chicken Salad with Avocado Dressing

Ingredient	Quantity	Instruction	Nutritional Information per Serving	Serving Size	Cooking Time
Chicken breast	2 pieces (6 oz each)	Grill until fully cooked and	High in protein, low in fat	1 serving	20 minutes

		slice thinly			
Mixed greens	4 cups	Rinse and dry	Rich in vitamins A, C, K, and fiber	1 serving	N/A
Cherry tomatoes	1 cup	Halve	Source of vitamins C and K, antioxidants	1 serving	N/A
Cucumber	1 medium	Slice thinly	Low in calories, provides hydration	1 serving	N/A
Avocado	1 whole	Blend with lemon	High in healthy	1 serving	5 minutes

		juice, salt, and pepper for dressing	fats, fiber		
Lemon juice	2 tablespoons	Mix into avocado dressing	High in vitamin C	1 serving	N/A

Instructions:

- Preheat the grill. Season the chicken breasts lightly with salt and pepper, and grill each side for about 10 minutes until fully cooked. Let it rest before slicing.
- Prepare the avocado dressing by blending the avocado with lemon juice, salt, and pepper until smooth.
- Toss the mixed greens, cherry tomatoes, and cucumber in a large bowl. Top with sliced chicken and drizzle with avocado dressing.

Cooking Time: Total preparation and cooking time is approximately 25-30 minutes.

Serving Size: Makes 2 servings.

Nutritional Information: Each serving provides a balanced mix of protein, healthy fats, and essential vitamins, making it suitable for those managing EPI, aiding in digestion and nutrient absorption.

2. Quinoa and Roasted Vegetable Bowl

Ingredient	Quantity	Instruction	Nutritional Information per Serving	Serving Size	Cooking Time
Quinoa	1 cup	Cook in 2 cups of water	High in protein, fiber, and essential minerals	1 serving	15 minutes
Bell peppers	1 cup sliced	Roast in the oven	Rich in vitamin C and	1 serving	25 minutes

		with a drizzle of olive oil	antioxidants		
Zucchini	1 cup sliced	Roast together with bell peppers	Provides vitamin C, potassium, and fiber	1 serving	25 minutes
Carrots	1 cup sliced	Roast together with other vegetables	High in beta-carotene and fiber	1 serving	25 minutes
Olive oil	1 tablespoon	Use for roasting vegetables	Healthy fats	1 serving	N/A

Fresh parsley	To garnish	Chop and sprinkle over the top	Vitamin K and antioxidants	1 serving	N/A

Instructions:

- Preheat the oven to 400°F (204°C). Toss the sliced bell peppers, zucchini, and carrots with olive oil and spread them out on a baking sheet. Roast in the oven until tender and slightly caramelized, about 25 minutes.
- While the vegetables are roasting, rinse the quinoa under cold water, then cook in boiling water for about 15 minutes until tender. Fluff with a fork.
- Assemble the bowl by adding a base of quinoa, topped with roasted vegetables. Garnish with chopped fresh parsley.

Cooking Time: Total preparation and cooking time is about 40 minutes.

Serving Size: Makes 2 servings.

Nutritional Information: This meal is rich in vitamins, minerals, and fiber, supporting digestive health and nutrient absorption. The protein from quinoa provides energy without stressing the pancreas, ideal for EPI management.

These lunch recipes provide practical, nutritious, and easy-to-prepare options for individuals managing EPI, helping to maintain a balanced diet while addressing specific digestive needs.

Dinner Ideas

Meal planning is key for individuals managing Exocrine Pancreatic Insufficiency (EPI), as it helps ensure that meals are balanced, nutritious, and minimize the risk of gastrointestinal distress. Here, we focus on dinner options that are tailored to be EPI-friendly, avoiding high-fat ingredients and difficult-to-digest foods. Each recipe includes a detailed breakdown of ingredients, instructions, nutritional information, serving size, and cooking time to help streamline meal preparation.

1. Baked Lemon Herb Chicken

- **Ingredients:** 4 boneless, skinless chicken breasts, 2 lemons (juiced), 1 tbsp olive oil, 1 tsp dried oregano, 1 tsp dried basil, salt and pepper to taste.
- **Instructions:** Preheat oven to 375°F. In a bowl, combine lemon juice, olive oil, oregano, basil, salt, and pepper. Place chicken in a baking dish and pour the mixture over the chicken. Bake for 25-30 minutes or until the chicken is cooked through.
- **Nutritional Information:** Each serving provides approximately 200 calories, 35g protein, 5g fat, 0g carbohydrates.
- **Serving Size:** Serves 4.
- **Cooking Time:** 30 minutes.

2. Quinoa and Vegetable Stir-Fry

- **Ingredients:** 1 cup quinoa, 1 cup chopped carrots, 1 cup diced bell peppers, 1 cup chopped zucchini, 1 tbsp olive oil, 1 tbsp low-sodium soy sauce, 1 garlic clove minced.
- **Instructions:** Cook quinoa according to package instructions. Heat olive oil in a skillet over medium heat. Add garlic, carrots, bell peppers, and zucchini. Stir-fry for about 5-7 minutes until vegetables are tender. Add cooked quinoa and soy sauce, stir well to combine.
- **Nutritional Information:** Each serving contains about 220 calories, 8g protein, 5g fat, 40g carbohydrates.
- **Serving Size:** Serves 4.
- **Cooking Time:** 20 minutes.

3. Grilled Tilapia with Mango Salsa

- **Ingredients:** 4 tilapia fillets, 1 ripe mango (peeled, pitted, and diced), 1/2 red bell pepper (diced), 1/4 cup chopped red onion, 1 tbsp chopped cilantro, juice of 1 lime, salt and pepper to taste.
- **Instructions:** Preheat grill to medium-high heat. Season tilapia with salt and pepper, and grill each side for 3-4 minutes until the fish flakes easily with a fork. In a separate bowl, combine mango, red bell pepper, onion, cilantro, and lime juice. Serve salsa over the grilled tilapia.
- **Nutritional Information:** Each serving offers approximately 180 calories, 23g protein, 2g fat, 15g carbohydrates.
- **Serving Size:** Serves 4.
- **Cooking Time:** 20 minutes.

4. Turkey Meatballs in Tomato Sauce

- **Ingredients:** 1 lb ground turkey breast, 1 egg, 1/4 cup breadcrumbs, 1/2 tsp garlic powder, 1/2 tsp onion powder, 2 cups low-sodium tomato sauce.
- **Instructions:** Preheat oven to 400°F. In a bowl, mix ground turkey, egg, breadcrumbs, garlic powder, and onion powder. Form into small meatballs and place on a baking sheet. Bake for 20 minutes. Heat tomato sauce in a saucepan and add cooked meatballs. Simmer for 10 minutes.
- **Nutritional Information:** Each serving includes approximately 240 calories, 28g protein, 10g fat, 12g carbohydrates.
- **Serving Size:** Serves 4.
- **Cooking Time:** 30 minutes.

These recipes provide a variety of dinner options that cater to the dietary needs of those with EPI, focusing on low-fat, easily digestible, and nutrient-rich ingredients. Planning meals around such recipes can help manage symptoms and ensure a balanced diet.

Snacks and Desserts

Meal planning for individuals managing Exocrine Pancreatic Insufficiency (EPI) requires thoughtful consideration of ingredients and preparation methods to ensure meals are both nutritious and easy to digest. This detailed plan covers three main meals—breakfast, lunch, and dinner—along with snack and dessert options that adhere to EPI dietary guidelines.

Breakfast: Low-Fat Blueberry Pancakes

Ingredient	Quantity	Instruction	Nutritional Information per Serving	Serving Size	Cooking Time
Whole wheat flour	1 cup	Use as base for pancake batter	High in fiber, iron	2 pancakes	20 minutes
Fresh blueberries	1/2 cup	Mix into batter	Rich in antioxidants,	2 pancakes	20 minutes

			vitamin C		
Low-fat milk	3/4 cup	Mix into batter to create desired texture	Provides calcium, vitamin D	2 pancakes	20 minutes
Egg	1	Add to batter for binding	High in protein, vitamins B12 and D	2 pancakes	20 minutes
Baking powder	1 tsp	Add for leavening		2 pancakes	20 minutes
Olive oil spray	To coat	Spray on skillet	Low in saturated fat	2 pancakes	20 minutes

Lunch: Grilled Chicken Salad

Ingredient	Quantity	Instruction	Nutritional Information per Serving	Serving Size	Cooking Time
Skinless chicken breast	6 oz	Grill until cooked through	High in protein, low in fat	1 serving	25 minutes
Mixed greens	2 cups	Use as salad base	Low in calories, high in vitamins	1 serving	25 minutes
Cherry tomatoes	1/2 cup	Halve and add to salad	Good source of vitamin C, potassium	1 serving	25 minutes

| Cucumber | 1/2 cup | Slice and add to salad | Hydrating, provides silica | 1 serving | 25 minutes |
| Low-fat vinaigrette | 2 tbsp | Dress salad | Low in calories | 1 serving | 25 minutes |

Dinner: Baked Salmon with Steamed Vegetables

Ingredient	Quantity	Instruction	Nutritional Information per Serving	Serving Size	Cooking Time
Salmon fillet	6 oz	Bake in oven at 350°F	High in omega-3 fatty acids, protein	1 serving	30 minutes

| Broccoli | 1 cup | Steam until tender | High in fiber, vitamin C | 1 serving | 30 minutes |
| Carrots | 1 cup | Steam until tender | Rich in beta-carotene, fiber | 1 serving | 30 minutes |

Snack: Greek Yogurt with Honey and Almonds

Ingredient	Quantity	Instruction	Nutritional Information per Serving	Serving Size	Cooking Time
Low-fat Greek yogurt	1 cup	Serve chilled	High in protein, low in fat	1 cup	0 minutes

| Honey | 1 tbsp | Drizzle over yogurt | Provides antioxidants, natural sugar | 1 cup | 0 minutes |
| Sliced almonds | 1 tbsp | Sprinkle on top | Good source of healthy fats, protein | 1 cup | 0 minutes |

Dessert: Baked Pear with Cinnamon

Ingredient	Quantity	Instruction	Nutritional Information per Serving	Serving Size	Cooking Time

| Pear | 1 medium | Core and slice | High in fiber, vitamin C | 1 serving | 30 minutes |
| Cinnamon | 1 tsp | Sprinkle on pear before baking | Anti-inflammatory, lowers blood sugar | 1 serving | 30 minutes |

These meals, snacks, and desserts provide balanced options that adhere to the dietary needs of individuals with EPI, focusing on low-fat, nutrient-rich ingredients that are easy to digest. The recipes are designed to minimize the risk of digestive discomfort while ensuring nutritional adequacy, making meal planning a supportive tool in managing Exocrine Pancreatic Insufficiency.

Conclusion

Managing Exocrine Pancreatic Insufficiency (EPI) requires careful consideration of diet and lifestyle, a journey that is both personal and unique to each individual affected by this condition. Through the guidance provided in this EPI diet food list, the goal has been to empower readers with the knowledge necessary to make informed decisions about what to eat and what to avoid. This understanding is essential in reducing symptoms, enhancing nutrient absorption, and improving overall quality of life.

Throughout the book, the emphasis on avoiding certain foods while encouraging others is more than just a list of dos and don'ts; it is a fundamental approach to managing a complex condition with dietary adjustments. Each section of this guide has been crafted to provide comprehensive insights into how foods interact with the body when EPI is present, offering alternatives that maintain a balanced and nutritious diet without causing additional stress to the pancreas.

The importance of adapting recipes and meal planning cannot be overstated. As illustrated in the recipes and meal suggestions included in this guide, each ingredient has been carefully selected to minimize the risk of exacerbating EPI symptoms. These adaptations not only cater to nutritional needs but also ensure that meals remain enjoyable and diverse, an important aspect of maintaining a healthy relationship with food despite dietary restrictions.

The discussion on hydration has highlighted another crucial aspect of managing EPI. Adequate fluid intake is vital for digestion and the effectiveness of pancreatic enzyme replacement therapy, a common treatment for EPI. By understanding the role of hydration in digestive health, individuals can better manage their condition and avoid complications associated with dehydration.

Social engagements and dining out are part of normal life, and this guide has aimed to equip readers with strategies to handle these situations without fear. Knowing how to choose appropriate foods from a menu and how to communicate dietary needs to others can greatly reduce the anxiety associated with eating in social settings. This empowerment is essential for maintaining social connections and quality of life.

Keeping a food diary as recommended can serve as a powerful tool for managing EPI. By tracking what you eat and how it affects your body, you can gain deeper insights into your personal triggers and better tailor your diet to suit your specific needs. This proactive approach is crucial in managing a chronic condition like EPI, where small adjustments can make significant differences in how you feel.

In conclusion, this guide has provided a roadmap for navigating the dietary challenges posed by Exocrine Pancreatic Insufficiency. With careful consideration and adaptation, it is entirely possible to lead a fulfilling and healthy life despite the constraints of EPI. The journey is continuous and may require adjustments along the way, but with the right tools and knowledge, each individual can find their own path to wellness.